Chronically Stoned

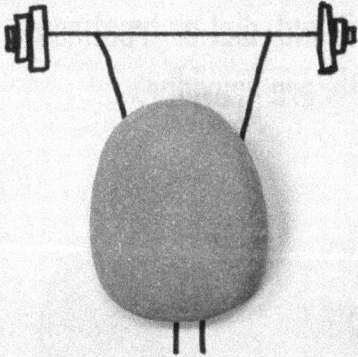

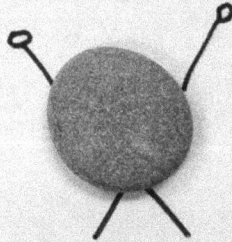

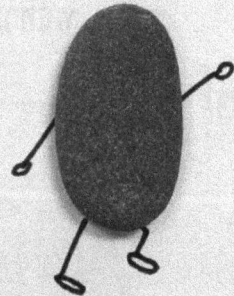

Guide to winning the battle against kidney stones.
By: Winslow E. Dixon

This book was written as a guide on how to fight the battle against kidney stones and urinary tract infections from the patient perspective of Winslow E. Dixon; a chronic kidney stone former and sufferer of Medullary Sponge Kidney (Cacchi-Ricci Disease).

-DISCLAIMER-

The information in this book is not to be used to
diagnose or treat any condition or to replace medical care.
Do not start or stop any medication, supplement, diet or treatment
without first contacting your healthcare provider.

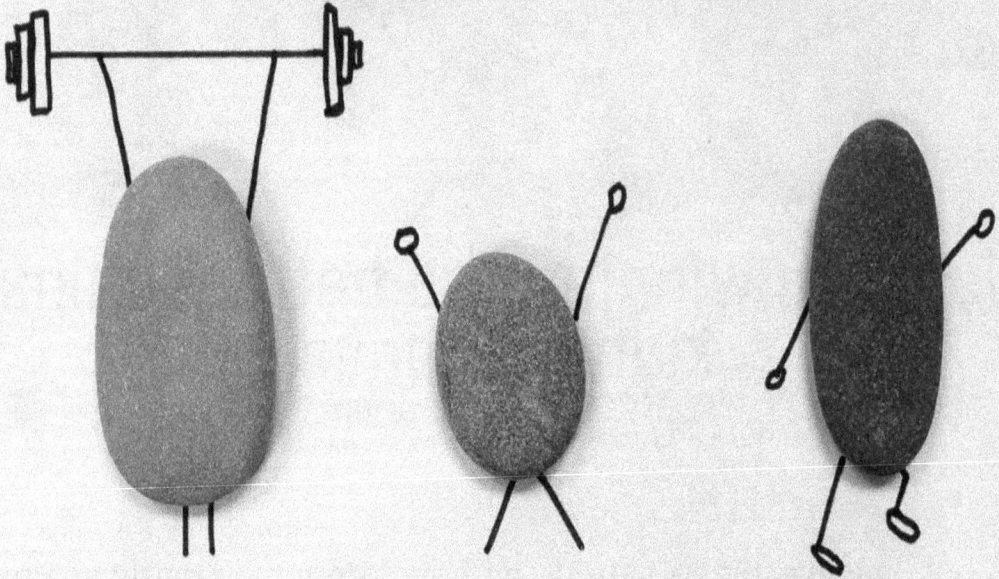

All comments, opinions and suggestions in this book were derived from the
patient perspective of Winslow E. Dixon.

If you are reading this, you are probably one of the lucky people who suffers with kidney stones. First of all, let me say I am sorry but you are not alone.

I wrote this book to share the information I have discovered to help conquer the very intense war against kidney stones, urinary tract infections and renal issues.

My name is Winslow E. Dixon. I have had kidney stones almost every single day since I was fifteen years old. I have a congenital disease called medullary sponge kidney (Cacchi-Ricci Disease) which causes me to have constant kidney stones, flank pain, renal colic and recurrent infections.

I know battling kidney stones can feel impossible, but I assure you it is not.

As someone who has passed thousands of kidney stones and suffered with countless urinary tract infections, I've learned many things in my quest to have quality of life despite my own health. I have written this book to share the information I've learned. It is my hope that the tips and tricks in this book will help others find hope, healing and happiness- even if you are chronically stoned!

This is your life.

This is your health.

You can take control.

You may have kidney stones, but they don't have you!

Thank you for reading, <u>Chronically Stoned</u>.

Now, let's get your quality of life back!

Table of Contents

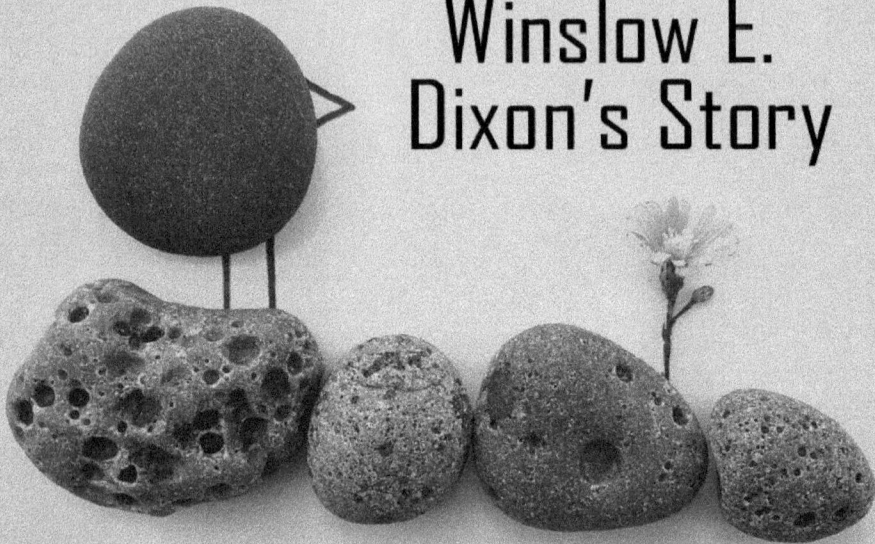

Winslow E. Dixon's Story

Winslow grew up in the American south in the state of North Carolina. She was your typical American kid. She loved to dance, sing and was full of life. She was an extroverted personality and always enjoyed being around people. She had dreams of being in the medical field and wanted to live her life serving others. But at age fifteen, she started having health problems. She suffered with frequent infections and started having chronic kidney stones. Winslow already suffered from migraines and endometriosis, but these new symptoms were different. What in the world could be causing this much pain?

Winslow continued to live life as normal as possible and suffered through every kidney stone and infection. Coupled with her other health issues, she started to struggle in school. After she passed out at school one day, her family decided to homeschool her. She continued her studies and was pleased to no longer be forced to attend school. The other kids didn't understand chronic pain and unfortunately the teachers didn't either. She graduated early and headed off to college.

Her first year of college proved to be a massive health challenge. Her freshman year she not only suffered with kidney stones but also had gallstones. A stone lodged itself in the bile duct and she was forced to have emergency surgery to remove her gallbladder. While she was in surgery, her appendix ruptured. In a weird yet miraculous way, the gallstones had saved her life. The surgeons also discovered she had aggressive endometriosis and a month later had a second surgery to remove it. All while this was happening, her kidney stones and infections did not stop. She went to emergency rooms repeatedly and was dismissed as a "seeker." With the recurrent infections, doctors accused her of being promiscuous.

Though she was a virgin, she was branded a drug seeking, loose young woman. They offered her no pain relief and no options. They convinced her it was all in her mind.

"There is no way possible one person can pass that many kidney stones." They told her.

In the small Carolina town, she was branded as a "seeker" and it got to the point where no one would treat her. She began to grow sicker and sicker. Her health failed completely. The physical stress of the chronic pain caused her to develop another disease- adrenal failure. Her body produced so much cortisol (the stress hormone) for so many years that it simply gave out. Her endocrine system completely failed. Winslow almost lost her life on her 23rd birthday when she suffered an adrenal crisis. She was later diagnosed with Addison's Disease.

Once again, amidst the other health issues, the kidney stones and infections did not stop. There had to be a reason for the pain she was feeling. Winslow decided she wouldn't give up until she found answers.

She sought the help of a hospital clinic based in Florida. She was referred to the "top kidney stone doctor." He ordered an MRI, blood work and urine tests. After all his testing, he told her there was nothing he could do and he had no diagnosis.

"Drink more water and try lemon juice." He told her.

Dismayed, she walked away feeling hopeless. Then she asked to be referred to another physician. She heard the clinic employed a "female urology specialist."

The "top stone" doctor reluctantly referred her care to the female doctor.

"I can refer you, but she won't tell you anything different than I just did, ma'am." He told her.

"That's fine. I just feel in my heart I need to try." Winslow replied.

Three months later she saw this female doctor. She was a kind woman of Indian descent. She reviewed her medical charts and pulled the imaging up on the computer screen at the appointment.

"You have something called Medullary Sponge Kidney." She told her. She then explained all the symptoms MSK caused. It was as if she had read Winslow's mind.

Finally, there was a name to the monster that plagued her for so long.

"Now that we know what this is- we can fight it. I am referring you to pelvic floor therapy, pain management and we will start you on medication to help you manage this disease." The kind doctor explained. Tears welled up in both the eyes of Winslow and her mother who had accompanied her to the appointment. Finally, answers had come. At 24 years old, Winslow was officially diagnosed with bilateral Medullary Sponge Kidney disease. She slowly started to learn how to manage both the Addison's disease and MSK.

Winslow wrote this book to share the tips that have helped her manage her chronic kidney disease. Her hope is that this book will help you manage your kidney issues and regain your quality of life.

Understanding Kidney Stones

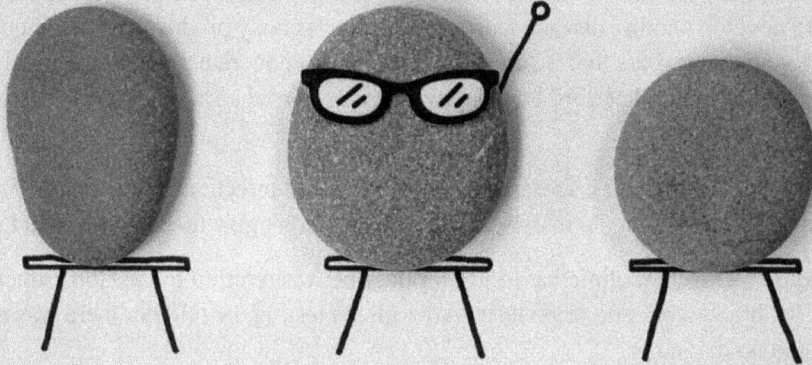

The National Kidney Foundation estimates that one in ten people will have a kidney stone at some time in their lives. Kidney stones are one of the top ten reasons that people visit emergency rooms.

Odds are, if you are reading this, you are one of the lucky people who suffer from chronic kidney stones. Let me first say that I am sorry. You are not alone. My hope is that you find some relief from the tips in this book.

The first step in kidney stone management is understanding what type of kidney stones your body makes and why.

Basic types of stones-

(Disclaimer- These are basic explanations of the most commonly formed kidney stones. For a complete list of kidney stone types, please consult your urologist for more information.)

Calcium stones- (Oxalate & Phosphate Stones) These are the most common form of kidney stones, usually in the form of calcium oxalate. Oxalate is a naturally occurring substance found in certain foods and is also made by your liver. Calcium stones may also be formed from calcium phosphate. This type of stone is more common in patients with chronic metabolic conditions such as **renal tubular acidosis** *(condition where the kidneys fail to properly acidify urine.)*

Struvite stones- These stones form due to urinary tract or kidney infections.

Uric acid stones- This type of stone typically forms in patients who are dehydrated and are more prevalent in people who eat a high-protein diet. People with gout also have increased risk of creating this type of stone. Genetic factors also may increase the risk of uric acid stones.

Cystine stones- This type of stone is found in people with a hereditary disorder that causes the kidneys to excrete too much of certain amino acids (cystinuria).

If you collect a stone that you've passed, your doctor can run a lab order to have it analyzed. This will tell you what your stones are made of and help you figure out the source. It is imperative you know what type of stone your body creates. You cannot battle something you don't fully understand.

Possible Kidney Stone Symptoms-

*(Disclaimer- This is not an all-inclusive list of all possible symptoms.
If you feel you may have a kidney stone, please consult your physician.)*

Flank pain
Radiating, sharp stabbing pains
Blood in the urine (red, pink, or brown urine)
Nausea
Vomiting
Discolored, cloudy or foul-smelling urine
Fever/Chills
Frequent urination
Renal colic

Everyone is unique and can experience different symptoms. If you suspect you are having kidney stones, straining your urine can help you determine if you are passing stones.

In addition to large stones, I also personally suffer from "kidney gravel" which are small, calcium phosphate stones that can be as small as a grain of sand. These stones cause me to have chronic pain, renal colic and frequent infections because my urinary tract is constantly being irritated. I did not discover this until I started to strain my urine.

It sounds gross, but it will help you understand what is going on with your body. I highly recommend having frequent urinalysis testing and straining your urine if you are suffering with renal and urinary symptoms.

Possible Causes of Kidney Stones-

*(Disclaimer- This is not an all-inclusive list of all possible causes for renal stone formation.
For more information please consult your physician.)*

There are many different reasons why people develop kidney stones. For me personally, I create kidney stones because the tubules in my kidneys did not form properly in the womb. I create calcium phosphate stones because my kidneys cannot adequately filter urine. Mine is a genetic source. My MSK causes a secondary diagnosis of renal tubular acidosis; which is when the kidneys fail to appropriately acidify the urine, creating an abnormal PH level.

Another genetic cause of kidney stones is found in those who have cystine stones due to a hereditary disorder that causes the kidneys to excrete too much of certain amino acids (cystinuria). There is conflicting research on whether there is a genetic predisposition for patients to become kidney stone formers or not. It differs on the type of stone and reason for onset. Some people have stones without a family history and others come from a long line of stone formers.

Other factors that can lead to Stone Production-

(Disclaimer- This is not an all-inclusive list of all possible reasons for renal calculi. For more information, please consult your physician.)

High doses of vitamin D
Gastro-intestinal bypass surgery
Disorders such as renal tubular acidosis and hyperparathyroidism
Metabolic disturbances
Low urine volume
Dehydration
High body mass index (BMI)
Diets that are high in protein, sugar and/or sodium
Digestive disorders

Again, everyone is different and may not have the same triggers. People with genetic factors have a hard time managing kidney stones because they are not caused by an external problem such as a diet triggers or dehydration.

Research says that a higher body mass index can increase the risk of stone production. In my own personal life, I suffered with stones when I was underweight, at an appropriate weight and also when I was overweight. This is why it is important to keep a journal of all your symptoms, what you eat and your lifestyle and environmental factors. You and your doctor will have to figure out if your kidney stones are genetic or caused by other factors.

Once you figure out what stones you make and why, you can begin a treatment plan.

Finding the right treatments and medication for you will not happen overnight. It will be a trial and error process but don't lose hope. There are thousands of medications and treatments available. There is something out there that can help you. I almost gave up complete hope before my diagnosis, but eventually found things that helped me manage my condition.

Additional Testing-

(Disclaimer- This is not a complete list of all possible tests for renal health. For more information, please consult your physician.)

Blood tests for calcium, phosphorus, uric acid, electrolyte levels, blood urea nitrogen (BUN), glomerular filtration rate (GFR) and creatinine levels to assess kidney function.

Urinalysis to check for crystals, bacteria, blood and white cells.

24 Hour Litho-Link Urine Test.

There are also imaging tests that can determine if you have lodged or embedded stones.

Additional testing may include: Abdominal X-rays, intravenous pyelogram (IVP), renal ultrasound, MRI or CT scan.

Emergency Room Concerns

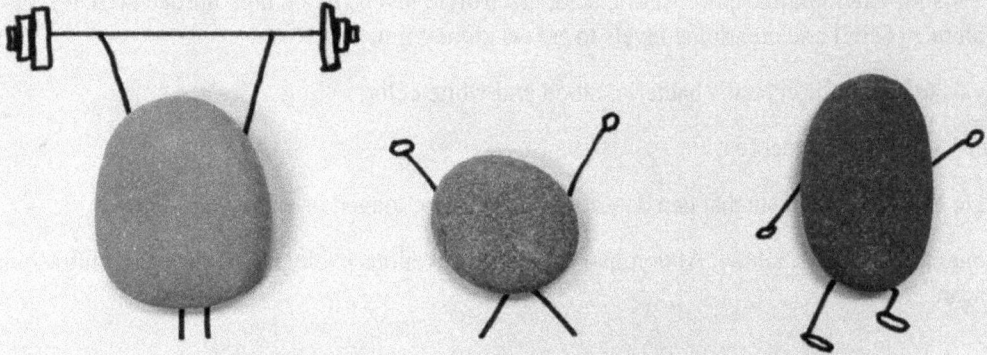

Visiting the emergency room can be a very daunting process. It is often packed with irritable people who are in pain, sick and impatient. Making the decision to go to the emergency room is something that chronic pain patients often ponder.

"Do I need to go to the emergency room or should I just suffer at home?"

This question is one only you can answer. But let me just caution you with the things I have learned.

The emergency room is purposed to handle traumatic situations such as car wrecks, heart attacks and broken bones. It is for the treatment of acute situations and not a place for extensive diagnostics. The doctors, nurses and care staff are trained to handle acute situations. I am not saying diagnostics do not happen in the emergency department, but for the most part the staff is trained to quickly assess, treat and clear the room for the next acute situation.

The emergency room is great for acute situations, but in my experience, they are not typically interested in figuring out anyone's extensive health puzzle. Their objectives are to stabilize a patient, make sure they are not in a critical, life-threatening state and discharge them.

Kidney stones are a horrific, painful experience. They are one of the top ten reasons people visit the emergency room. Kidney stones become life threatening when they become obstructed. The emergency department staff are trained to handle life threatening situations quickly, but pain management is not the main concern of emergency room staff.

Deciding whether to go to the emergency room or not is something you have to decide for yourself.

Check your vitals-

Heart rate

Blood pressure

Oxygen saturation rate

Respirations

This can help you decide whether or not you need medical intervention.

First line kidney stone treatment protocol is typically, **push fluids and manage pain**.

The emergency department may or may not give you pain medication for your kidney stones. This choice is dependent on the physician treating you. Some are more compassionate that others. Some believe kidney stones only hurt when they are moving or obstructive.

You know your body, if you feel that you are in need of medical intervention, please don't hesitate to visit the emergency room.

Just don't go in with the mindset of diagnostics, this is not the purpose of the emergency department. This is why finding a good urologist or nephrologist is essential to treating your kidney issues. They can spend time with you at your appointments and are not in a rush to clear a bed for an acute patient. These doctors can run extensive diagnostic tests to help discover how to better help you.

Finding a Good Doctor

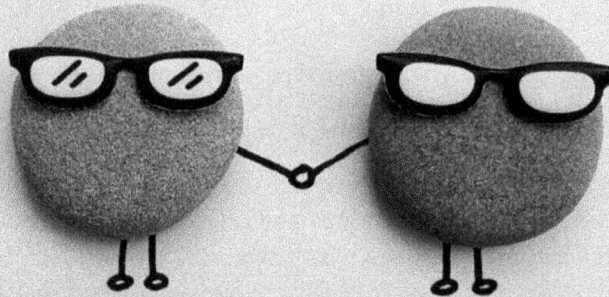

Finding a good doctor willing to help you is essential in managing your chronic kidney condition. I searched for years before I found a doctor who finally diagnosed me with medullary sponge kidney disease.

I had a doctor once tell me, "Everyone has crystals in their urine" and "It is impossible for someone to produce that many kidney stones." I was fortunate to finally find the doctor who diagnosed me and helped me manage my disease.

You deserve to find the right doctor who will not only treat your symptoms but validate you as a patient.

Do not accept "no" for an answer. There are countless urologists and nephrologists practicing medicine. You can find one that is willing to help you manage your health issues. Don't be afraid to "fire" a doctor that isn't helping you. This is your life, your body and your disease. You deserve to find answers. Don't give up until you find the proper care you deserve.

Reach out to online support groups for referrals. Social media can be a great resource to find people who may share your condition or symptoms. You can connect with people all across the world who may share in your hardships. Other patients may help direct you to the right doctor. I will just caution you to not use the internet to replace medical advice and to disengage if support groups become a source of stress. Social media can be a great resource; just be sure you are selective in who you interact with and never replace your medical care with social media suggestions.

Do your "homework." Have personal copies of your medical record and send them to the doctor before your appointment. This will give the physician a chance to understand your case and form a plan of action for treatment. According to the National Institutes of Health research, doctors only spend an average of fifteen minutes with each patient. It is difficult to explain your entire health history and form a proper treatment plan in such a short time period. Giving your doctor a "heads up" will give them a chance to fully understand your case. This will give you the best chance of managing your illness. When the doctor has a full understanding, they can better formulate a plan for you.

Advocate for yourself. If you are in pain, be honest about it. If you are constantly passing stones, let your doctor know. If you are struggling, don't suffer in silence. Don't be afraid to tell the truth. A good doctor will want to help you and not label you as a drug seeker.

Keep track of your symptoms. Keep a daily journal of your symptoms, the foods/beverages you ingest and the amount of sleep you're getting. Get a full picture of your own health so you can work with your doctor to eliminate things such as dietary or environmental triggers.

Surgical Interventions

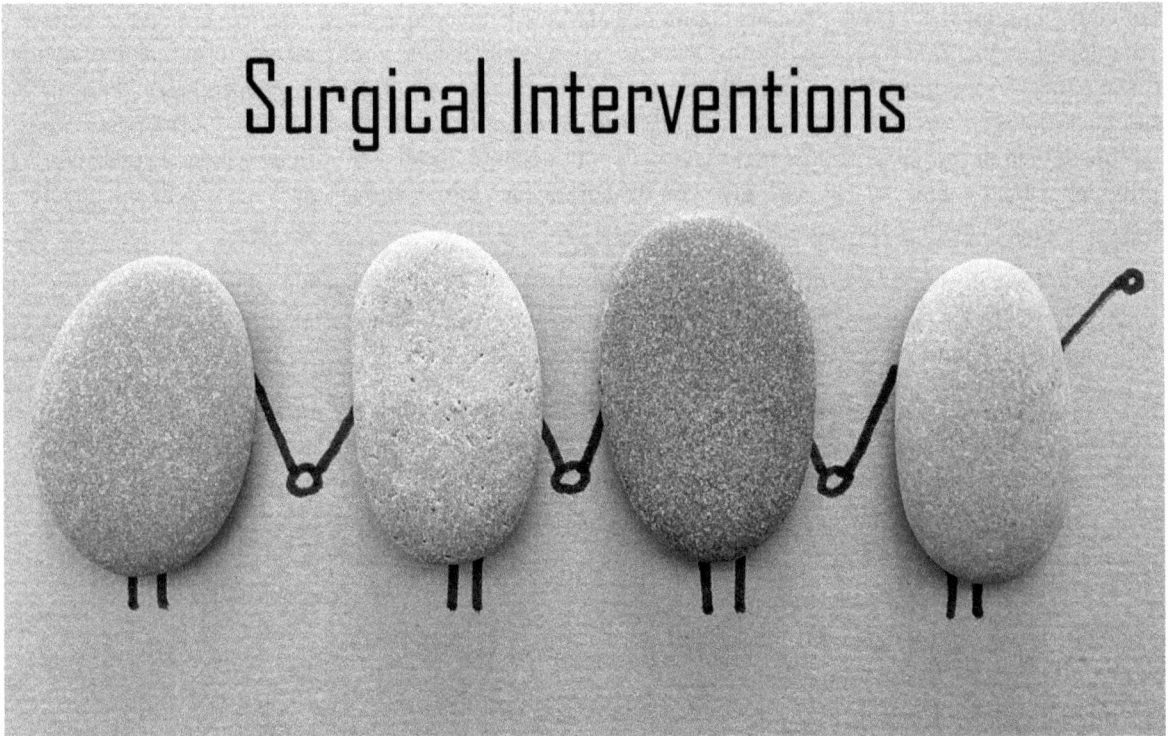

Unfortunately, sometimes kidney stones require surgical interventions if they do not pass naturally. This is not an inclusive list of all procedures used to treat renal issues but may be a suggestion to bring up to your physician.

Possible Surgical Options-

(Disclaimer- This is not a complete list of all possible surgical options.
For more information, please consult your physician.)

Shockwave lithotripsy- A common procedure performed under general anesthesia where sound waves are focused on renal calculi, resulting in the breaking of the stone(s) into small fragments. The stone fragments are then excreted through the urine.

Cystoscopy- A procedure where your doctor examines the lining of your bladder and urethra by using a hollow tube called a cystoscope. This tube is inserted into your bladder and can be used to diagnose bladder issues such as interstitial cystitis, tissue damage or stones in the bladder.

Ureteroscopy- A procedure where a scope is inserted through the urethra, bladder and into the kidney for removal of ureteral stones. The surgeon grabs the stone and removes it from the kidney or ureter. This is typically an outpatient procedure.

Percutaneous Nephrolithotomy- A procedure where the surgeon makes a small incision in the back, then by using a nephroscope (a miniature fiberoptic camera) removes the stone.

During most of these procedures, **a ureteral stent** is typically placed. This stent is a thin tube inserted into the ureter placed to prevent or treat obstruction of the kidney(s).

Though the stents are typically placed under general anesthesia, they are usually removed in the doctor's office without sedation. This sounds like a terrifying experience but let me assure you, it is far less painful than a kidney stone.

Before your stent removal, take your prescribed pain medications, hydrate and relax. The procedure only takes a few minutes and is tolerable. It sounds far worse than it actually is. I assure you, the pain of stent removal is nowhere near the pain of a kidney stone. Take heart that stent removal is nothing to be afraid of and is over in mere moments.

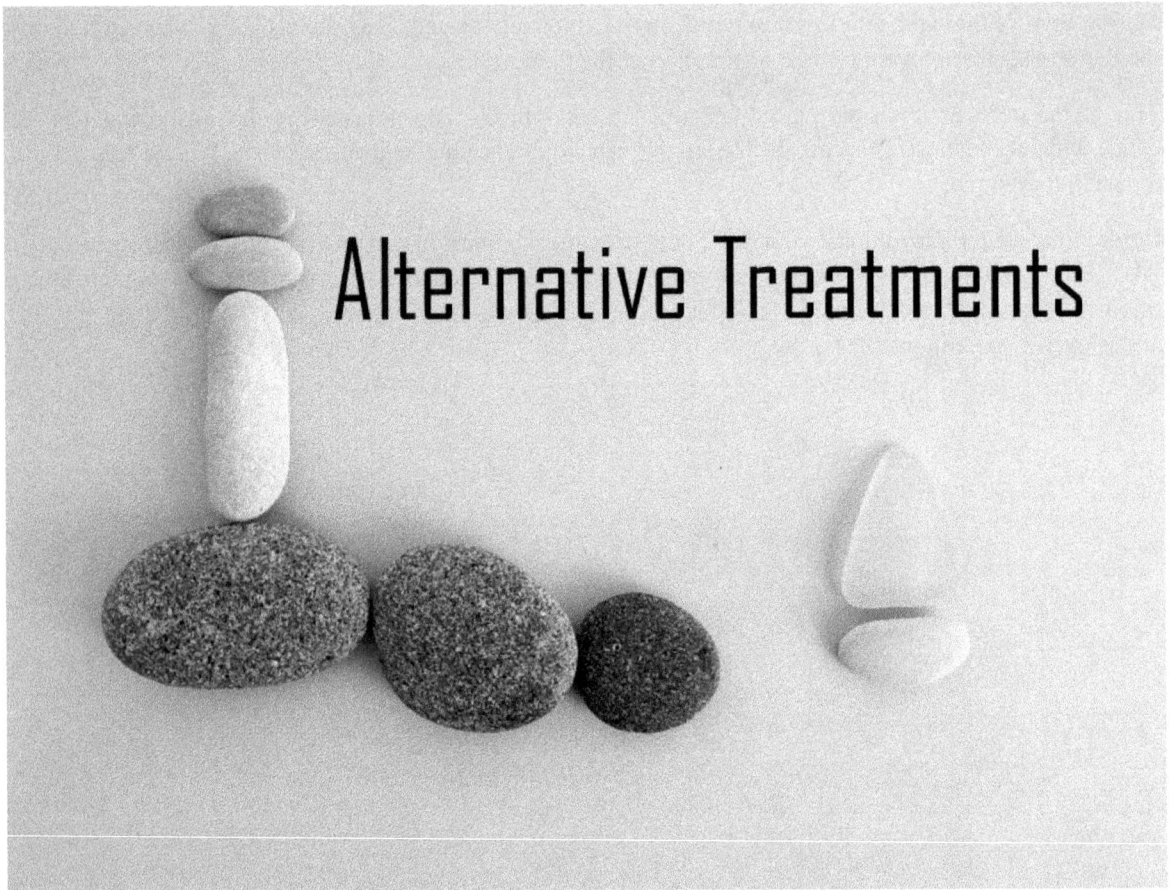

Alternative Treatments

The first line of treating kidney stones is to **eliminate the source**. If you discover that you are making stones that are triggered by certain diet choices, you must then eliminate those foods.

Example- A 20-year-old male body builder suddenly develops sharp flank pain after starting a high protein diet in addition to weight lifting classes. He visits the local emergency room to discover he has a kidney stone. He is referred to urology and given a urine strainer to catch his stone upon passing. Upon examination, the urologist determines his stones were caused by the excess protein in his diet. The patient is instructed to reduce the amount of protein in his diet to reduce his risk of stones.

With me personally, I found that citric acid was a major trigger for my renal colic and made my stone production much more intense. I constantly make stones, but when I ingested anything that had citric acid in it, my stones were much larger and my renal colic was much worse.

(Disclaimer- Do not start or stop anything without first contacting your healthcare provider. This is a patient perspective and a personal opinion; not to be used to replace or provide medical care.)

But why? Citric acid? Isn't that just lemons?

Come to find out, most citric acid is not made from lemons. It is derived from mold.

Citric acid is derived from **aspergillus niger**, which is a form of black mold.

Commercially produced citric acid is made by manipulating sugars exposed to black mold and filtered using sulfuric acid, which is a genetically modified organism (GMO).

Citric acid used to be made from fruit, but corporations found a cheaper short-cut by producing the GMO form. Unfortunately, this is now the common practice.

I am already allergic to penicillin, so my body does not like anything derived from mold. Eliminating citric acid from my diet took my daily pain levels from 8-10 to a manageable level. I still pass stones and have "bad kidney days" but I can honestly say I am not in 24/7 agony like I was.

Be vigilant about what goes into your body.

Read every label.

Ask questions.

Drink adequate water.

If foods are triggering your symptoms, eliminating them may help you have less pain.

Keep a daily journal to discover your dietary triggers.

Patients who develop stones due to unbalanced PH levels may find relief by eliminating acidic foods such as tomato sauce, peppers and acidic fruits like pineapple or strawberries. (*This is a patient perspective and a personal opinion; not to be used to replace or provide medical care.*)

Certain stones form in alkaline urine, while others form in acidic urine.

Stones that form in alkaline urine:

Struvite (magnesium ammonium phosphate)

Calcium phosphate

Stones that form in acidic urine:

Uric acid

Cystine

Calcium oxalate

Determining your specific stone formation and properly balancing your PH levels may help you manage your symptoms.

Everyone is different. You must learn what hurts you. Don't be afraid to be picky. If you can make your life better by eliminating certain foods, it is worth it.

As much as I love spaghetti sauce, I always regret eating it when my renal colic flares. Learning what triggers your symptoms can help you manage your pain.

Non- Medicinal Treatments-

*(Disclaimer- This is not a complete list of all possible non-medicinal options.
For more information, please consult your physician or holistic health practitioner.)*

Heating Pad- My heating pad is like my best friend. They have many types of these wonderful things. I have a vibrating heating pad that helps me pass the kidney gravel. It helps with flank pain as well. If you have kidney pain, get one of these. It's worth every penny. Be sure to never fall asleep on it and always be vigilant of the heat settings to prevent burns. Use extra caution if you are diabetic or on blood thinning medication.

Frequency Specific Microcurrent (FSM) Machine- This is an alternative therapy that I discovered at a holistic clinic. It is a device that uses frequency specific microcurrent waves (thus the acronym FSM machine). Basically, there are wave links that are programmed to impact certain parts of the body through "protocols." The FSM machine has many other protocols for pain, injury and relaxation. It sounds really "hippie" but it absolutely works. I went for treatment three times a week and eventually bought my own machine. It works by the principle of biologic resonance. Even the world-renowned Cleveland Clinic has adopted this method of alternative therapy. I highly recommend it. (Links to FSM treatment located in the source section of this book.)

Pelvic Floor Therapy- Passing chronic kidney stones can cause a lot of physical problems. Chronic urinary tract pain can lead to other issues such as voiding dysfunction and interstitial cystitis. PVT can help treat these issues. People with chronic kidney stones are also prone to develop chronic back pain due to the tendency to "tense" up from the pain of stones. Physical therapy can help you relax those tense muscles and help eliminate trigger points and spasms. Most insurance will cover this if your doctor refers you.

Aqua Therapy- Exercising with chronic pain can feel like an impossible task. Water therapy is a great way to exercise in way that causes less pressure on your joints, muscles and frankly your whole body. Movement has been researched to help stone passage. This is a great way to get moving in a gentle, low impact environment.

TENS Unit- (Transcutaneous electrical nerve stimulation) A machine that uses electrical current pulses produced by a device to stimulate the nerves for pain relief. To use, you simply place the electrode pads on the affected area and turn the frequency to a comfortable pulse. It is believed to help release the tension caused by chronic pain by calming the nerve impulses.

Essential Oils- There are various essential oils used for various things such as pain management and detoxification. There are many licensed holistic practitioners and aromatherapists that can help you discover which EO's are right for you. (Example-Peppermint oil applied topically is a natural pain reliever.)

As great as these non-medicinal options are, they sometimes are not enough to manage all symptoms of a kidney disease. Though they helped me, I still needed medicine for my MSK disease. I have passed hundreds of kidney stones; all the exercise in the world couldn't make that pain any less. Passing stones is a horrible painful experience. I also get frequent kidney infections and have interstitial cystitis. These are also painful. I require medication to help me cope with this pain.

"But you are SO YOUNG! You shouldn't be on medicine so young!"

Let me tell you the dangers of unmanaged pain. As you previously read in my story, I suffered for years before anyone would ever help me. I passed kidney stones, had endometriosis and migraines. I continued to work and be in school. I pushed myself through way too much pain for way too long.

Cortisol is the body's stress hormone. The body releases it in response to stress, pain and illness. My body produced so much cortisol for so many years that one day it just gave out. Now, I not only suffer from MSK but also have adrenal insufficiency; which is the lack of cortisol production caused by total adrenal failure. I truly believe that had my MSK been diagnosed earlier, I wouldn't have developed total adrenal failure.

Unmanaged pain is not something the body was created to handle 24/7.

There is such a stigma currently about the so-called, "opioid epidemic." I am all for the idea that doctors should try to treat the source of pain instead of masking it with medication. But the truth is, sometimes narcotic medications are necessary for quality of life. I am talking about proper use of this class of medications- to treat incurable, chronic pain.

Properly used opioids are not used to get high, they are used to give quality of life to those suffering with incurable, chronic pain or injury.

It is wrong that people say, "Opioids kill." Opioid ABUSE is what kills, not proper use of the medication used to treat incurable pain.

If you have chronic pain, don't suffer needlessly. There is no shame in becoming a pain clinic patient. This does not mean you are an addict. This just means you need help managing a painful condition. I don't want anyone to suffer the fate I now have unnecessarily. If you have unmanaged pain, please contact a physician.

That being said, narcotics are not the only medicines on the market. There are many classes of medications that can aid in the fight against kidney stone pain and discomfort.

Medications & Supplements

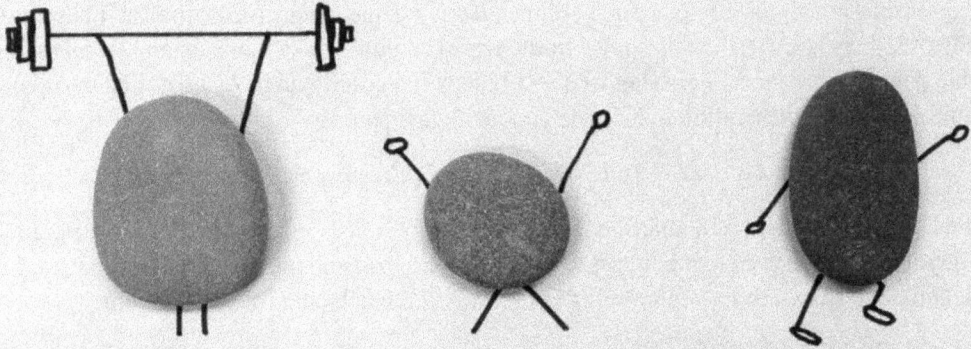

(Do not start or stop any medications, supplements or treatments without first consulting your physician. This information is only to be used as a patient's perspective and not to be used to treat or diagnose any condition. Contact your doctor regarding the use of any medications or treatments. This list is not to be used to replace medical advice.)

Medications-

(Disclaimer- This is not a complete list of all medications. For more information, please consult your physician.)

Ditropan (generic name- oxybutynin)- Antispasmodic and anticholinergic medication used to treat symptoms of overactive bladder but also found to be beneficial in patients with renal colic.

Levsin (generic name- hyoscyamine)- Antispasmodic medication beneficial in quelling renal colic and bladder spasms.

Atarax (generic name- hydroxyzine)- Antihistamine medication used to reduce pain and inflammation.

Elavil (generic-amitriptyline)- Tricyclic antidepressant medication used to reduce pain and may also help those suffering from depression due to chronic pain.

Elmiron (generic name- pentosan polysulfate sodium)- Mildly blood thinning medication that also works as a bladder protectant and is prescribed to treat bladder pain and discomfort.

Flomax (generic name- tamsulosin hydrochloride)- Alpha-blocker medication that relaxes the urinary tract, making it easier to urinate and pass stones. *(Be careful if you have a sulfa allergy if considering this medication.)*

Utira-C Tablets (generic name- hyoscyamine, methenamine, methylene blue, phenyl salicylate, sodium biphosphate)-Prescription medicine that contains multiple medications used in combination to treat urinary pain, spasms and inflammation.

Pyridium (generic name-phenazopyridine)- Analgesic medication used for relief of pain, burning and urgency of the lower urinary tract.

Natural Supplements-

(Disclaimer- This is not a complete list of all possible natural supplements. For more information, please consult your physician or holistic health practitioner.)

IP-6 Inositol- A vitamin-like substance found in seeds that has been reported to prevent the formation of kidney stones. It is also used as an immune support and cancer fighter.

Chanca Piedra- An herb believed to relieved to aid in dissolving kidney stones, increase urine output and have activity against bacteria and viruses, also believed to help lower blood sugar. (Diabetics and people with hypoglycemia should use this with caution.)

Oregano Oil or Capsules- Oregano is a natural antimicrobial and can be used to prevent infection caused by kidney stones.

Marshmallow Root- Natural herbal anti-inflammatory used to lessen the inflammation in the urinary and respiratory tracts. Can be ingested in the form of capsules, powder or made into a warm tea.

From my personal experience, I had a grand benefit from Elavil. It helped reduce my chronic pain immensely. I have personally been on all these medications/supplements and they have helped me. That being said, **EVERYONE IS DIFFERENT**. You and your doctor can figure out what treatments work best for you.

Something else that helped me greatly were bladder instillations. My urinary tract typically stays very inflamed from the impact of the constant kidney gravel. Bladder instillations helped me reduce my pain levels.

Bladder instillations are performed by inserting a catheter into the bladder and filling it with a combination of medications to treat the symptoms of burning pain or interstitial cystitis. The combination is inserted into the bladder and the patient "holds" the liquids for as long as possible. The medications reduce inflammation and discomfort within the bladder. A urologist can prescribe this treatment and it is an outpatient procedure, usually performed by a nurse.

You can suggest any of these treatments to your doctor. Not all things work for everyone, but hopefully you will be able to find some relief from at least one of the previously mentioned medications, treatments or natural remedies.

Urinary Tract Infections

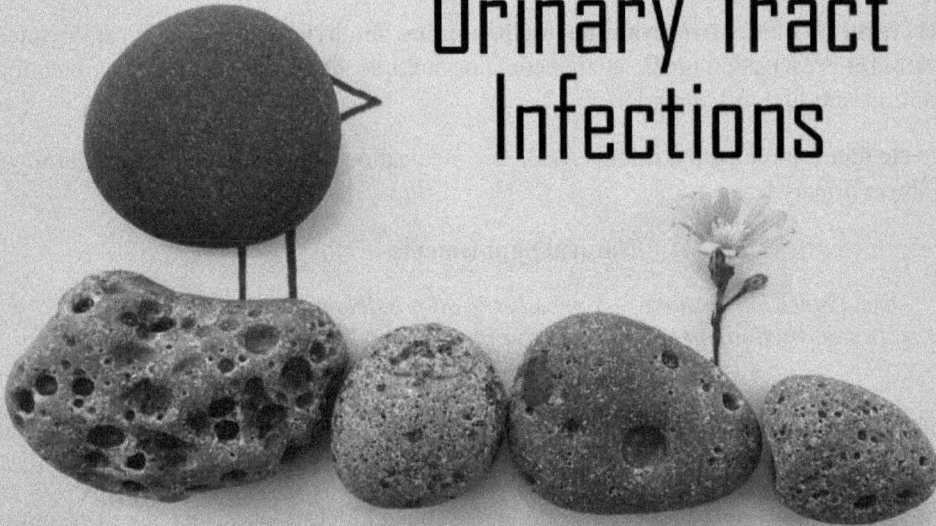

Patients who struggle with kidney stones are at increased risk to develop urinary tract infections. If you are a chronic UTI sufferer, it is imperative you get frequent urinalysis testing with your physician. At home PH test strips can also be beneficial to assessing whether infection is present. These at home tests may not be as accurate as clinical testing so it is important to communicate with your healthcare provider if you are exhibiting symptoms. Again, everyone is unique and can experience different symptoms. If you suspect you have a UTI, call your doctor.

Possible Symptoms of UTI-

(Disclaimer- This is not an all-inclusive list of all possible symptoms, please consult your physician for more information.)

Fever, shaking and/or chills
Nausea
Vomiting
Bladder pain (cystitis)
Pelvic pressure
Lower abdominal discomfort
Painful urination
Blood in urine
Burning with urination
Frequent urges to urinate

Antibiotics

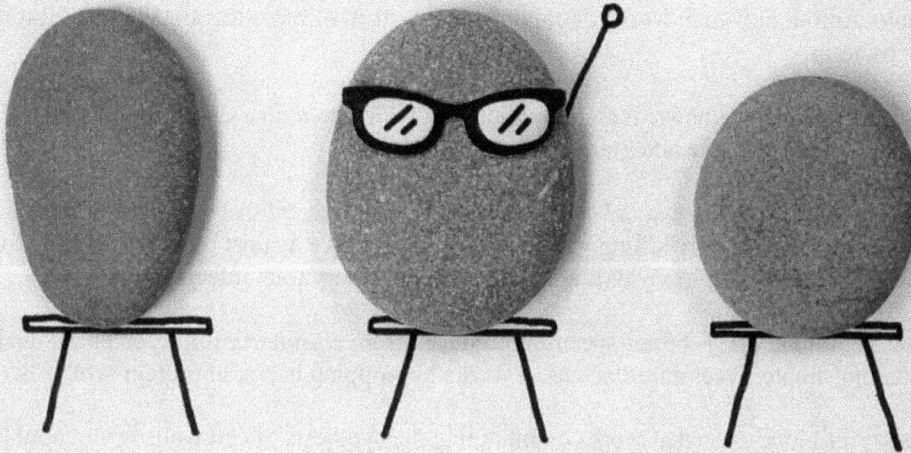

Antibiotics are typically the first line treatment in managing urinary tract infections. It is important to completely finish your antibiotic treatment to completely eradicate the infection. Antibiotic resistance can occur if you abruptly stop treatment before the full course of antibiotics have been administered.

Antibiotic resistance- The process of bacteria mutating to the point it inhibits the effectiveness of medications used to treat infections; therefore, causing the antibiotics to be ineffective in curing infections.

Types of Antibiotics-

(Disclaimer- These are basic explanations of antibiotics from a patient's perspective, not to be used to replace medical care or advice.)

Penicillins- Antibiotics derived from *penicillium fungi,* which work by preventing the cross linking of amino acid chains in the bacterial cell wall.

Cephalosporins- Antibiotics derived from the mold, *acremonium*. They work by binding and blocking the activity of enzymes responsible for making *peptidoglycan-* a component of the bacterial cell wall.

Macrolides- Antibiotics derived from *streptomycetes*, a type of bacteria found in soil that makes the decomposition of plants possible. They work by binding to the bacterial ribosome and inhibiting bacterial protein synthesis.

Lincosamides- Antibiotics which include lincomycin, clindamycin, and pirlimycin. They work by preventing bacteria from replicating by interrupting the synthesis of proteins.

Sulfonamides- Antibiotics made from *sulfanilamide*, a sulfur-containing chemical. This class of antibiotics works by preventing the production of *dihydrofolic acid*, a form of folic acid that bacteria and human cells use for producing proteins.

Nitroimidazole- Antibiotic which works through the mechanism of bioreduction and to inhibit infection by killing the bacteria.

Quinolones- Antibiotics also known as fluoroquinolones, which contain a fluorine atom and are effective in the treatment of gram-negative and gram-positive bacteria.

Nitrofurantoin- Antibiotic class that is *bacteriostatic,* a chemical agent that stops bacteria from reproducing, while not necessarily killing it. Nitrofurantoin is active against gram positive organisms and is also used to treat females as prophylaxis against recurrent urinary tract infections.

Tetracyclines- Antibiotic that is broad-spectrum produced from *chlortetracycline*, an antibiotic isolated from the bacterium streptomyces aureofaciens. It works by stopping bacterial protein synthesis.

Glycopeptides- Antibiotic class that works by inhibiting the synthesis of cell walls in susceptible microbes. They are narrow spectrum in use because they only affect gram positive bacteria. This class of medication is understood to be used as a "last resort" drug in human medical practice because of its possible toxicity.

Aminoglycosides- Antibiotics derived from *streptomyces griseus,* a species of bacteria found in soil which enact bactericidal activity against gram-negative aerobes and is commonly used in the treatment of serious infections caused by aerobic gram-negative bacilli.

Carbapenems- Antibiotics which work by killing bacteria by binding to penicillin-binding proteins and preventing bacterial cell wall synthesis. A benefit to this class of medications is that they are commonly unaffected by antibiotic resistance. These medications contain broad spectrum of activity and potency against gram-positive and gram-negative bacteria. According to the National Center for Biotechnology Information, this class of drugs is used as "last-line agents" or "antibiotics of last resort."

Treatment Concerns

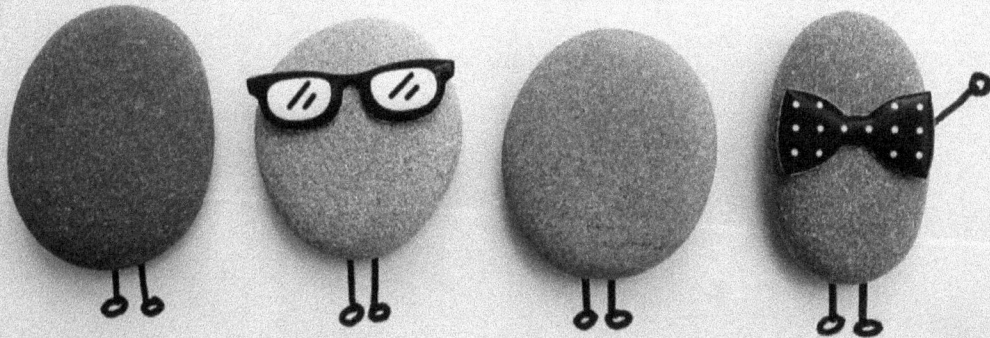

Antibiotics are beneficial in the management of urinary tract infections but can also cause secondary issues such as candida, C-diff infections and antibiotic resistance.

Candida- An overgrowth of fungus that occurs when the PH balance in the body is disrupted and can be caused by antibiotic, oral contraceptive or corticosteroid use. Using probiotics in addition to your antibiotics may prevent you from developing candida.

Possible Symptoms of Candida-

(Disclaimer- This is not a complete list of all possible symptoms, for more information please consult your physician.)

Sugar Cravings
Exhaustion
Bad breath
White Coating on Tongue
Hormonal Imbalance
Joint pain
Low Libido
Allergies
Gas/Bloating
Weakened Immune System

The treatment for candida is typically oral anti-fungal medications, probiotics and eliminating sugar from your diet. If you suspect you are suffering from candida, contact your healthcare provider.

Clostridium difficile (C-diff)- Occurs when the healthy bacteria in the colon is disrupted, often from the use of antibiotics. Though the C. diff bacteria is commonly found in soil, water and feces; it is a contagious infection and can cause colon damage.

Possible Symptoms of C-Diff-

(Disclaimer- This is not a complete list of all possible symptoms.
For more information please consult your physician.)

Abdominal cramping
Fever
Nausea
Loss of appetite
Weight loss
Diarrhea
Dehydration
Rapid heart rate

If you are having any of these symptoms, consult your doctor. They can order the diagnostic tests to determine if you have an active C-diff infection. You will have to provide a stool sample for testing and your doctor can determine if you need further treatment.

The treatment of C-diff are medications such as metronidazole, vancomycin
fidaxomicin which are commonly used in the management of this issue. In extreme cases, surgical interventions are also used if colon damage has occurred.

Sepsis

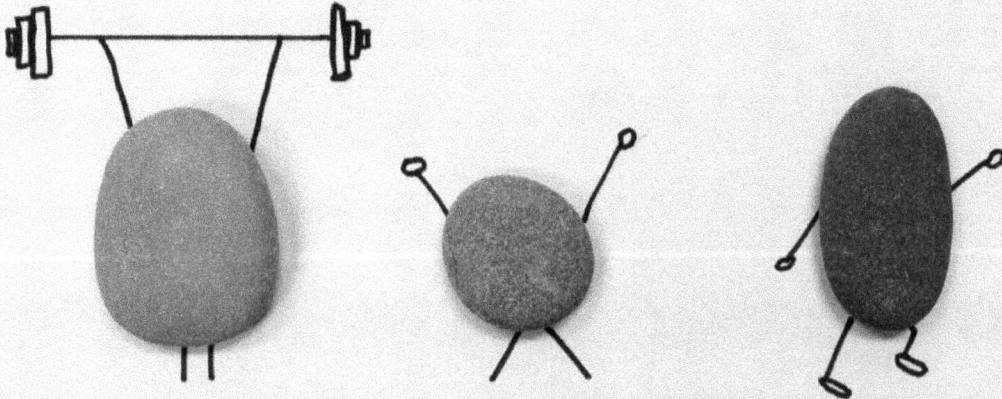

Sepsis- When infections, bacteria or germs enter a human body and are not properly treated it can cause sepsis. Septic shock has a fifty percent mortality rate; which is why urinary tract infections must be addressed with timely and appropriate treatment.

Possible Symptoms of Sepsis-

(Disclaimer- This is not a complete list of all possible symptoms.
For more information please consult your physician.)

Confusion or disorientation
Temperature changes such as fever at or above 100°F or a temperature below 96.8°F
Heart rate higher than 90 beats per minute
Breathing rate higher than 20 breaths per minute
Probable or confirmed infection
Shortness of breath
Shivering or feeling very cold
Extreme pain or discomfort
Clammy or Sweaty Skin
Unconsciousness
Weakness

If you suspect you have a severe infection or could be septic, visit your local emergency room **immediately**. Sepsis can turn deadly, extremely quickly. This is why it is imperative to have frequent urinalysis testing if you are a chronic stone former.

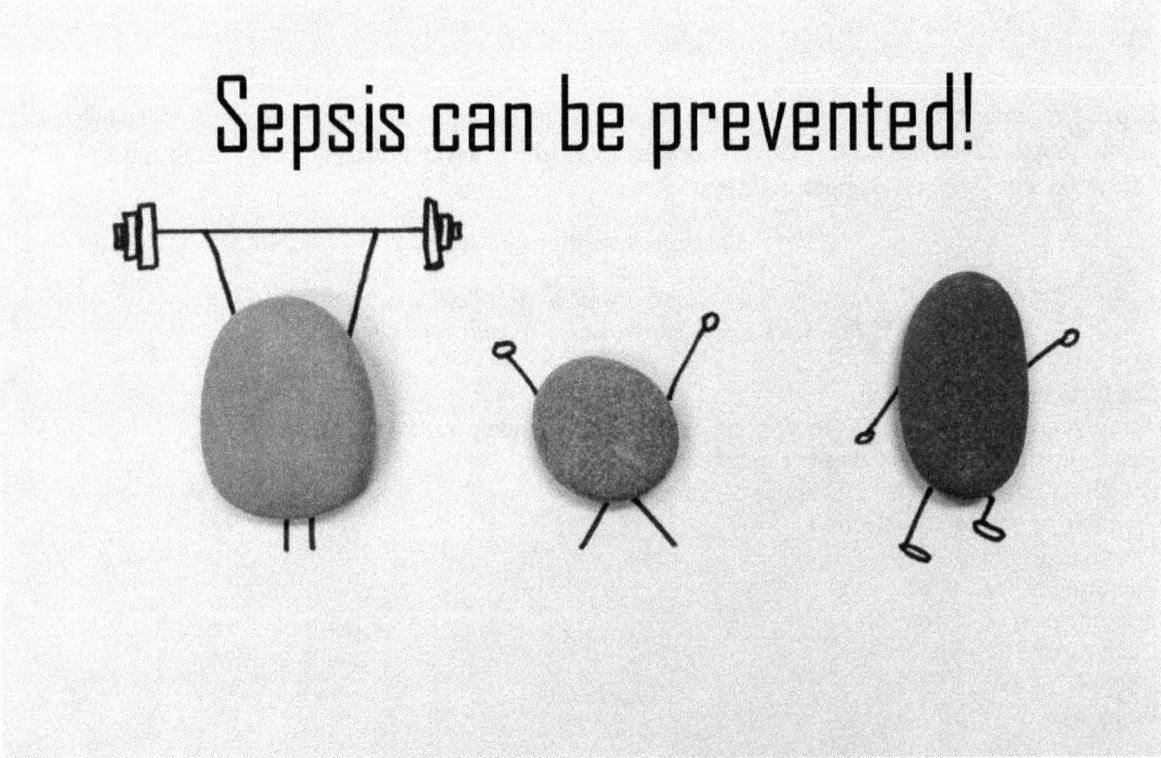

Sepsis can be prevented!

Preventing UTI's

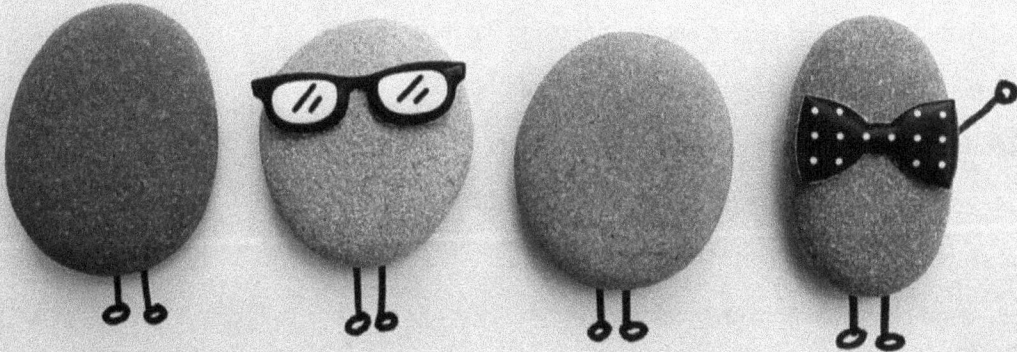

In chronic stone formers, the chance for contracting urinary tract infections is increased. There are many proactive steps you can take to prevent UTI's.

(The following suggestions are from a patient's perspective and are not to be used to replace medical care. Do not start or stop any medications, treatments, diets or alternative therapies without first consulting your healthcare provider.)

Hydration- This is the first defense in preventing urinary tract infections. When you are dehydrated, your body does not have the proper fluid content to perform at optimal function. Dehydration can also lead to the formation of kidney stones. Do yourself a favor and drink an adequate amount of water every single day.

Oregano Oil or Capsules- Oregano contains active biological substances which researchers have discovered has the ability to stop bacteria from producing urease (a substance found in pathogenic bacteria.) Many studies have shown that oregano has some of the strongest urease-inhibiting phenols. Some patients have found when ingesting oregano oil or capsules they see a decrease in urinary tract infections.

D-mannose- A simple sugar derived from fruits and is naturally found in certain cells in the human body. This powder or supplement is used for preventing urinary tract infections. It works by inhibiting bacteria from bonding to the urinary tract, therefore preventing infections.

Vitamin C- A vitamin that has been researched to inhibit the growth of E. coli and enhances immune function. This vitamin can be taken daily and may help you reduce the amount of UTIs.

Additional Tips-

Urinate as you feel the need to.

If you are female- Use natural, unscented feminine products.

Use quality toilet paper and wipe properly after using the restroom.

Urinate after intimate contact and be sure to bathe afterwards.

Wear comfortable cotton undergarments in your proper size and change them daily.

Avoid staying in wet clothing such as bathing suits/swim trunks.

Practice proper hygiene and perineal care.

Take all your medications as prescribed.

Avoid excess sugar and eat nutritiously.

Emotional Effects

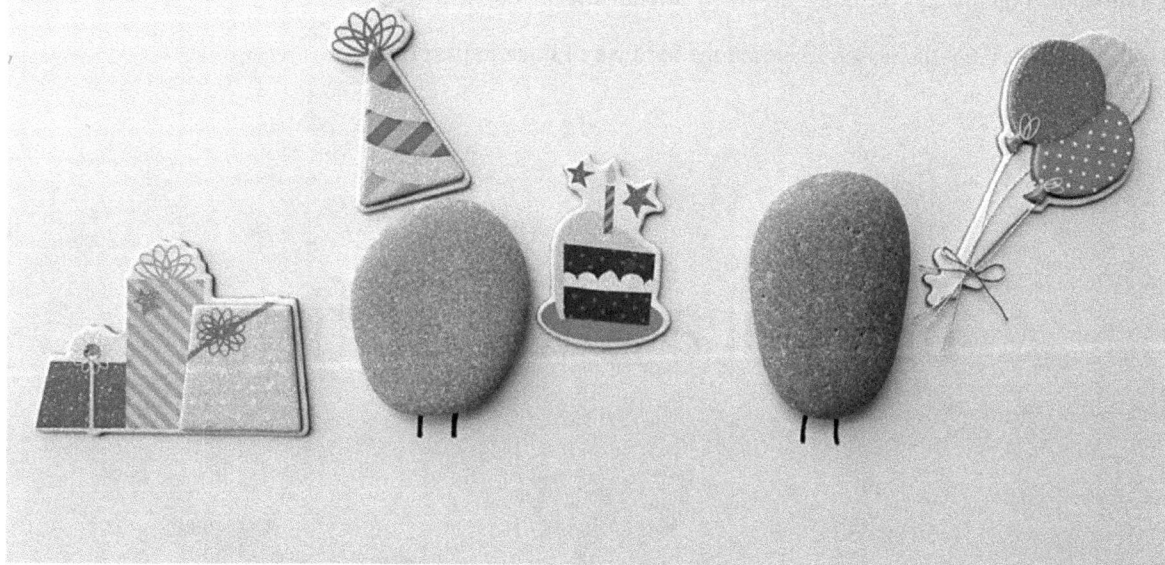

Finding treatments that work for you is essential to getting your quality of life back. I know firsthand the debilitating impact that chronic pain and illness can have on your life. Staying sane is half the battle when you are fighting a disease.

Most people do not understand that once health is lost, it takes just about everything with it. The inability to live your life the way you want to due to pain, fatigue and symptoms can depress even the strongest of people.

I knew at an early age I was never going to be a normal, healthy person. I did the worst possible thing you can do with any illness, I ignored it. I pushed myself through pain and fatigue. I worked in the healthcare industry in geriatrics (the elderly) as a MedTech. I worked in the nursing home setting. I can remember having to lay down in the floor of my patient's rooms to handle the pain. I would grit my teeth, rest for a second and fight back tears. I would pull myself together and then continue to give medications and care for my residents. I grew sicker and sicker until mind over matter didn't work anymore. I developed total adrenal failure (Addison's disease) because I didn't take care of myself.

At 24 years old, I was so unwell I couldn't even shower myself. My "mind over matter" mentality almost sent me to an early grave. The chronic kidney stones/infections coupled with the endometriosis and migraines caused too much stress on my body. Being a type "A" personality, I continued to push myself way further than my body could go. My mind was much stronger than my body was, and I almost led to my own demise.

Don't be like me. I am not saying you have to "*lay down and die*" and just accept your disease. But you do have to realize that you do have limitations.

You have to listen to your body's whispers for help before it starts screaming at you.

I believe my body produced so much cortisol for so many years that I absolutely burned my endocrine system out.

I almost died on my 23rd birthday due to an adrenal crisis.

Is this rare? Yes, but the lesson I learned the hard way I hope to pass on.

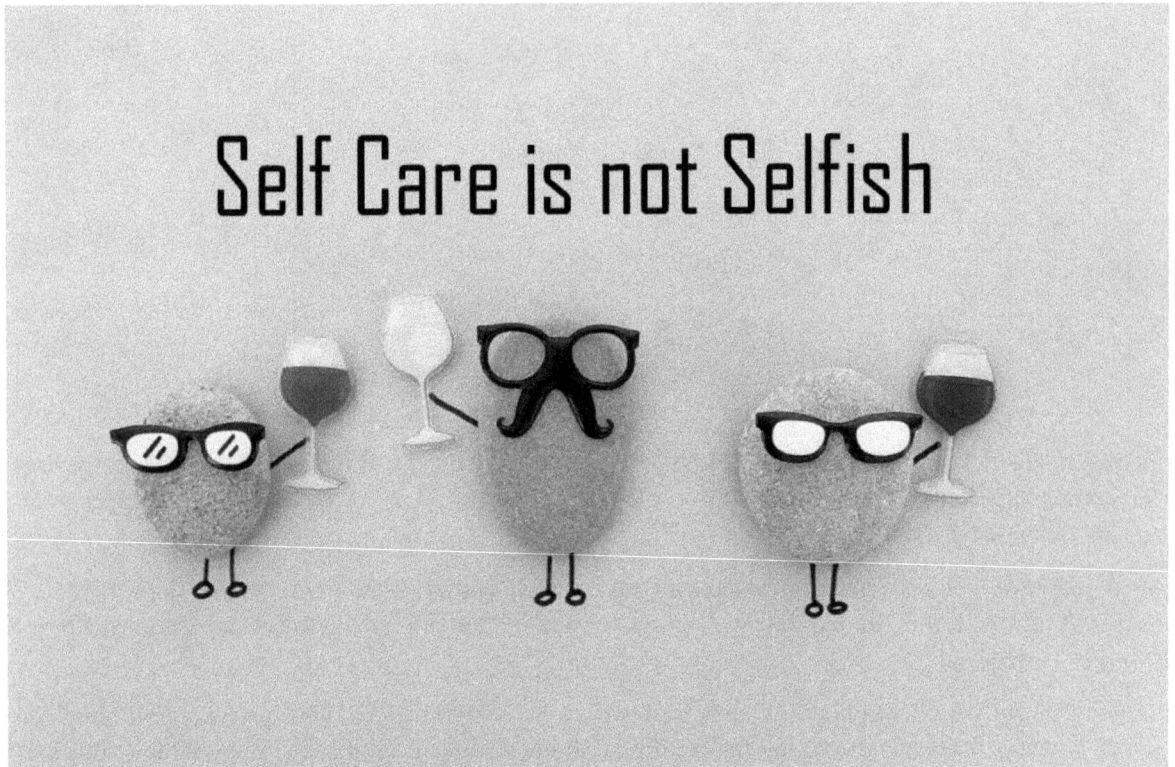

Self Care is not Selfish

There is no shame in resting if you need it.

There is no shame in taking medication.

There is no shame in taking care of yourself.

You are worth it!

Self- Care

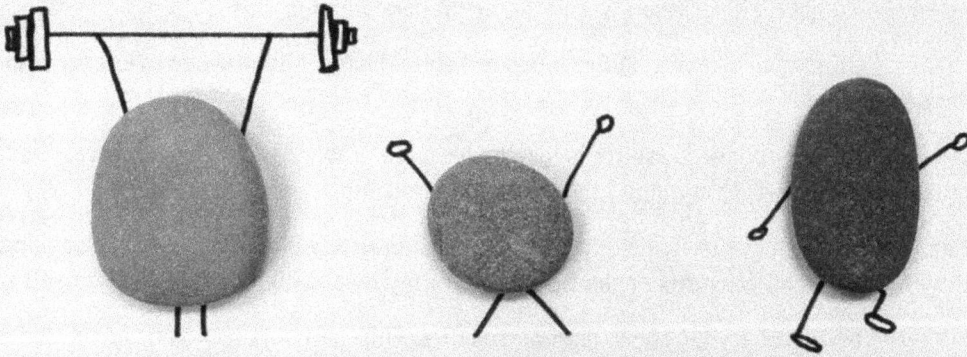

If you are depressed over your health, assess your life.

Ask yourself these questions-

Are you eating and hydrating properly?

Are you surrounding yourself with people who support you or tear you down?

Is your stress level high?

Are you doing things you enjoy?

Are you focusing on the negative or the positive in your life?

Are you getting enough sleep?

Is your life chaotic?

Are you making yourself a priority?

Self-care is not selfish!

Taking care of yourself is essential in any human life, but especially for those who suffer with health problems. You can't lift anyone else up with broken wings.

In my life, I neglected to take care of myself. I worked two jobs and was in school. I let my health get to a point it never should have, all because I wasn't taking proper care of myself.

I wasn't eating, hydrating or sleeping half as much as I should have. I didn't want to ask for help. I didn't want to burden anyone.

Fast forward in time, now I have to ask for help. I've been out of work and unable to drive, due to my health for the last two years. Everything I thought I was preventing I ended up causing.

At 24 years old, I had to move back in with my parents and basically became a child once again. I rely on them for my needs now all because I neglected to care for my own. You have to make yourself a priority.

No, I don't mean become a bratty "queen bee" personality. This does not mean you are entitled and can become bitter about your disease and your life. It simply means that you value yourself enough to give your body, soul and mind what it needs.

You cannot help anyone else if you have nothing left to give.

You can always get more money, a different job and material things; but once your health is gone it is not so easily obtained again.

Take Care of Yourself-

Drink enough water.

Eat the right foods.

Sleep at least eight hours a night.

Exercise at your tolerance level. Go for a walk.

Take your medication.

See your doctor.

Eliminate Stress.

Know your limits.

Listen to your body.

Keep track of your vitals.

Stay away from negative people as much as possible.

Make Yourself a Priority-

You have to become your own advocate. This is your life, your body and your disease. You have to do what is best for you. There is no shame in that. If someone shames you for that, that reveals their character and doesn't change yours. The people who truly care for you want you to be taken care of. They want you to practice selfcare. They want you to be well. If someone is constantly tearing you down, that is going to directly impact your health. Do not allow someone to make you feel guilty for things you cannot control. You didn't ask to have a disease. You didn't do anything to cause it so why would you take ownership and feel guilt over it?

Guilt is a useless emotion. You can't blame yourself for something you had no control over. Eliminate anyone in your life who is making you feel guilty over your own health. You are worth much more than that. You don't deserve to be treated that way. You've been through enough. Don't expose yourself to any more pain!

That being said, we can put guilt on ourselves as well. I did for many years. I felt like because I was sick I had to prove myself even more than the average person. I held back tears, got sick at work and school and pretended like I was fine. I hid the true reality of my health far too long to the point it forever damaged me. You don't have to do that. Kidney stones are horrifically painful. They can bring a grown man to tears. Give yourself a break.

Be Your Own Friend-

One of the most beneficial lessons I ever learned was to become my own friend. Your inner voice needs to be a positive one. You wouldn't constantly berate someone else for their shortcomings, why do you do it to yourself?

This is a habit I had to break. I used to break down into tears every time I showered because I would look at the destruction my body suffered due to my disease. I watched my once cute, slender female figure morph into a body that was scarred from surgery, steroid use and weight gain. I hated myself. I blamed myself for causing this. I thought if only I'd done everything differently I'd still be working, I'd still be beautiful, I'd still be....me....

But the reality is, disease can take a lot of things, but it can never take who you really are. Your character is revealed when all else is gone.

Don't beat yourself up because you can't do the things you want to do because of your disease or pain. Be your own friend. Care for yourself. Think positive thoughts about yourself.

Hating who you are isn't going to help you heal. It isn't going to change your situation for the better. It will only drag you into depression. Pain and illness are depressing enough, don't add self-hatred to the mix.

You are still you, despite any disease.

Replacing every negative thought with a positive one is a way to retrain your mind to be friendly. It becomes so easy to focus on the bad parts of our lives. When we switch our focus, our world seems much brighter.

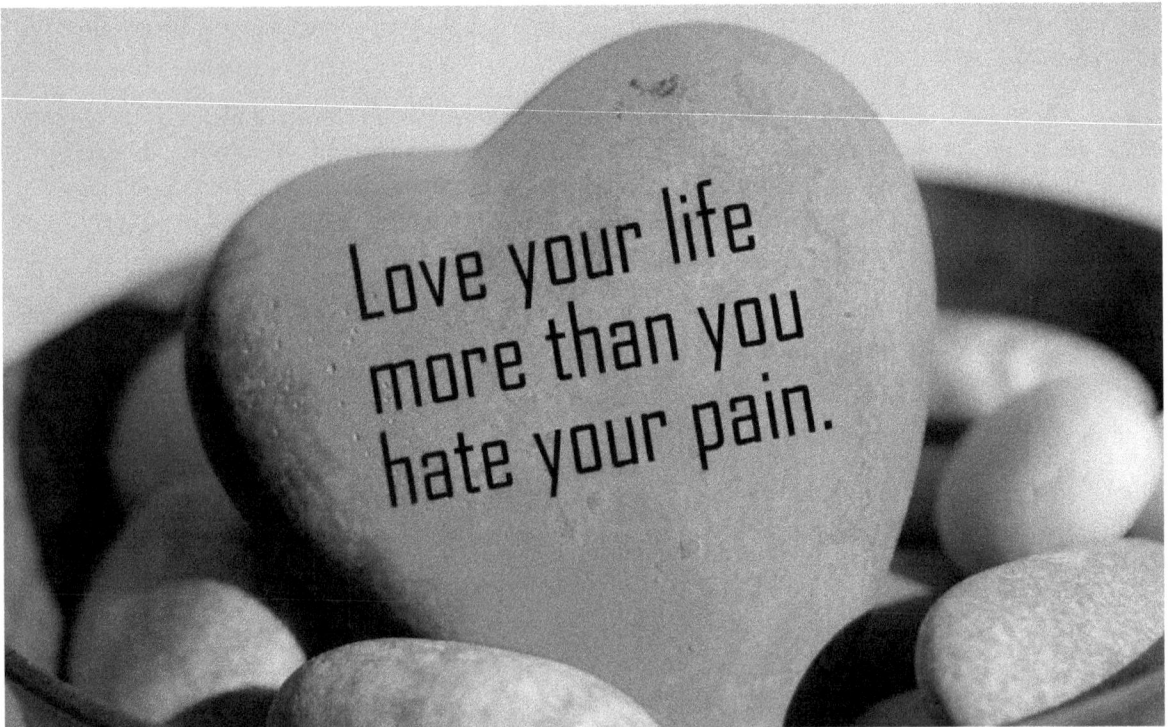

Plan of Action

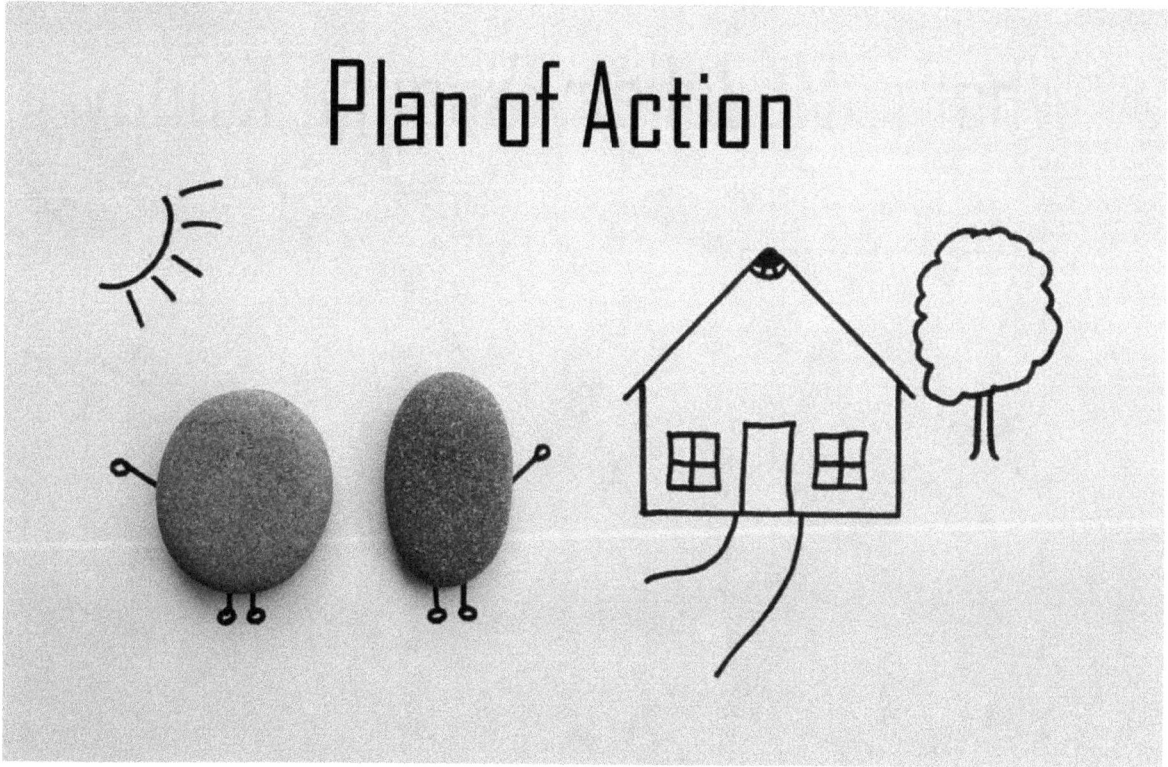

Plan of action when you are "chronically stoned"

1-Understand what types of stones you create.

2-Keep a daily log of your diet, lifestyle and symptoms.

3-Find a good doctor.

4-Get a plan of treatment. (Medications, dietary interventions, surgical options, physical therapy, supplements & alternative therapies.)

5-Make yourself a priority. (Practice self-care)

Chronic kidney stones can impact your life, but you cannot allow them to take control of your life. They may change your ability to live life the way you want to, but that does not mean you can't live a fulfilling existence.

You are still in control of your life. You can control what you eat, who you surround yourself with and your thoughts, actions and behaviors.

You may have kidney stones, but they don't have you.

What is Medullary Sponge Kidney

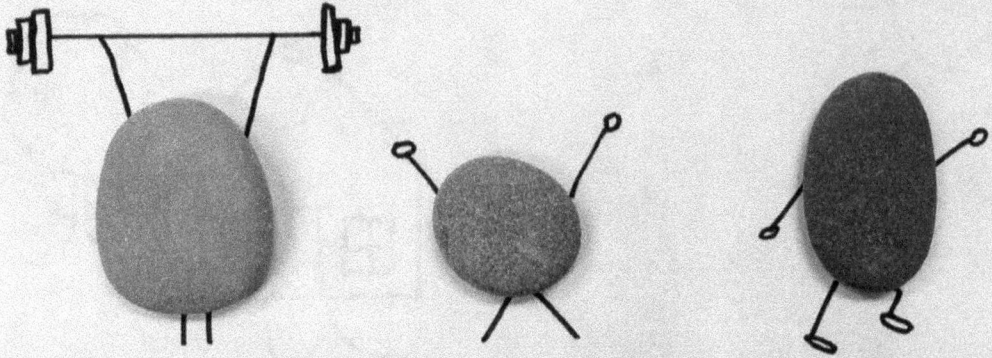

(The following information is from a patient's perspective and is not to be used to treat or diagnose any condition or to replace medical care. Do not start or stop any medications, treatments or alternative therapies without first consulting your healthcare provider.)

Although it only impacts a small amount of the population, I wouldn't feel right completing this book without mentioning Medullary Sponge Kidney (Cacchi-Ricci Disease).

This disease is the reason I have suffered with chronic kidney stones, renal colic, interstitial cystitis, and frequent, recurrent urinary tract infections most of my life. It is my belief that a great deal of chronic stone formers actually have MSK but are not tested for it.

Cacchi-Ricci Disease is primarily known as Medullary Sponge Kidney (MSK). It is a congenital disorder of the kidneys. Though it is present from birth, symptoms typically do not occur until adolescence. MSK occurs when the tubules in the kidneys do not properly form in the womb. This results in cystic dilations of the collecting tubules in one or both kidneys. On imaging scans, this shows up as a "sponge like" appearance. 70% of cases are bilateral, which means MSK occurs in both kidneys.

Patients with MSK are at increased risk for kidney stones and urinary tract infection. They typically pass twice as many stones per year as do other stone formers. Over 55% of MSK patients report chronic kidney pain, renal colic, frequent stones and recurrent infections.

MSK was previously believed not to be hereditary but there is more evidence coming forth that may indicate otherwise. There is conflicting evidence as to whether this condition is of genetic origin.

This kidney disease is unique because patients are, for the most part told they are not candidates for transplant. Though MSK can cause sub-par kidney function, only 10% of patients suffer renal failure and require dialysis. This disease, however is listed as one of the top painful conditions according to the American Chronic Pain Association. Sufferers of this disease complain of symptoms such as: Constant flank pain, renal and bladder spasms, pain associated with stone passage and frequent urination. Though not present in all cases, a common marker for this disease is the formation of "Kidney Gravel." These are small, sand-like stones that some MSK patients pass every single day of their lives. These grains cause frequent irritation in the urinary tract; which in turn causes pain, inflammation and leads to infection. This "sand paper" effect can also cause issues such as bloody urine, constant pain and interstitial cystitis in the bladder.

Diagnosis-

(This is not a complete list of diagnostic possibilities for Medullary Sponge Kidney, for more information please contact your healthcare provider.)

The standard diagnostic test most urologists use is called an intravenous pyelogram (IVP) An IVP is an x-ray examination of the kidneys, ureters and urinary bladder that uses iodinated contrast material injected into veins.

Blood tests for calcium, phosphorus, uric acid, electrolyte levels, blood urea nitrogen (BUN), glomerular filtration rate (GFR) and creatinine levels to assess kidney function.

Urinalysis to check for crystals, bacteria, blood, and white cells.

24 Hour Litho-Link Urine Test.

There are also imaging tests that can determine if you have lodged or embedded stones such as: Abdominal X-ray, renal ultrasound, MRI or CT scan.

Treatment-

(This is not a complete list of treatment possibilities for Medullary Sponge Kidney. For more information please contact your healthcare provider.)

Being a rare disease, the treatment for MSK can vary. Diagnostic tests such as urine PH and stone analysis can help sufferers discover what type of stones their body makes and why. Over 50% of MSK patients create calcium stones. Getting a urine PH test is essential to care with MSK because certain stones form in alkaline urine while others form in acidic urine.

Dietary interventions are beneficial in the management of this disease in addition to drinking adequate amounts of water.

Pain management is typically a necessary intervention in the treatment of MSK. Kidney stones are severely painful, and most patients need some sort of pain relief. Medications such as antispasmodics, urinary analgesics and narcotics can be prescribed to manage the agony of MSK. Pelvic floor therapy is also recommended.

No two people are the same and you should discuss all options with your urologist. Most patients require a combination of dietary changes, medications and physical therapy to manage medullary sponge kidney (Cacchi-Ricci Disease).

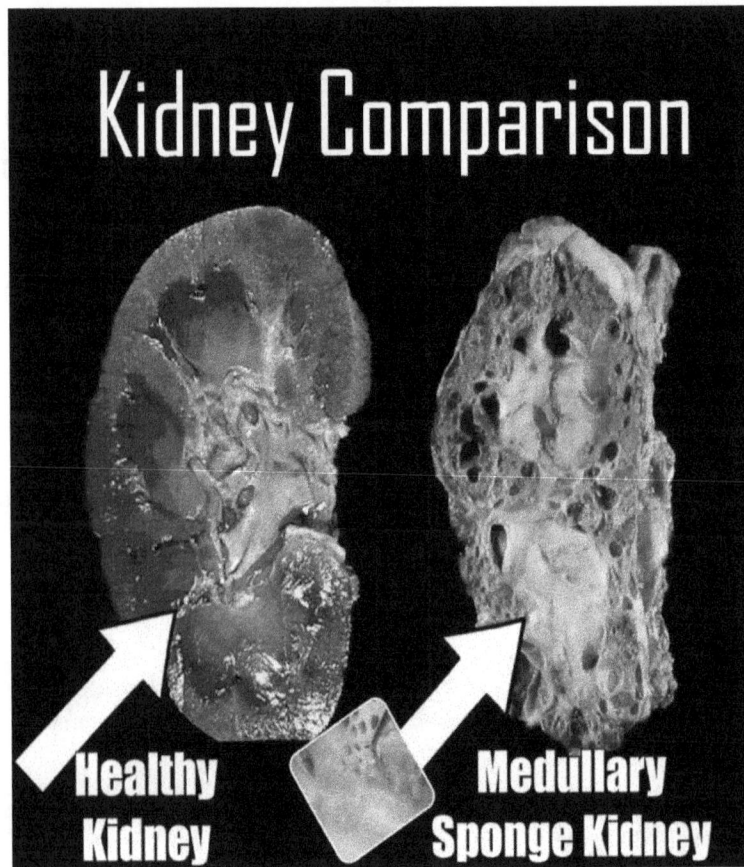

Kidney Comparison

Healthy Kidney

Medullary Sponge Kidney

Conclusion

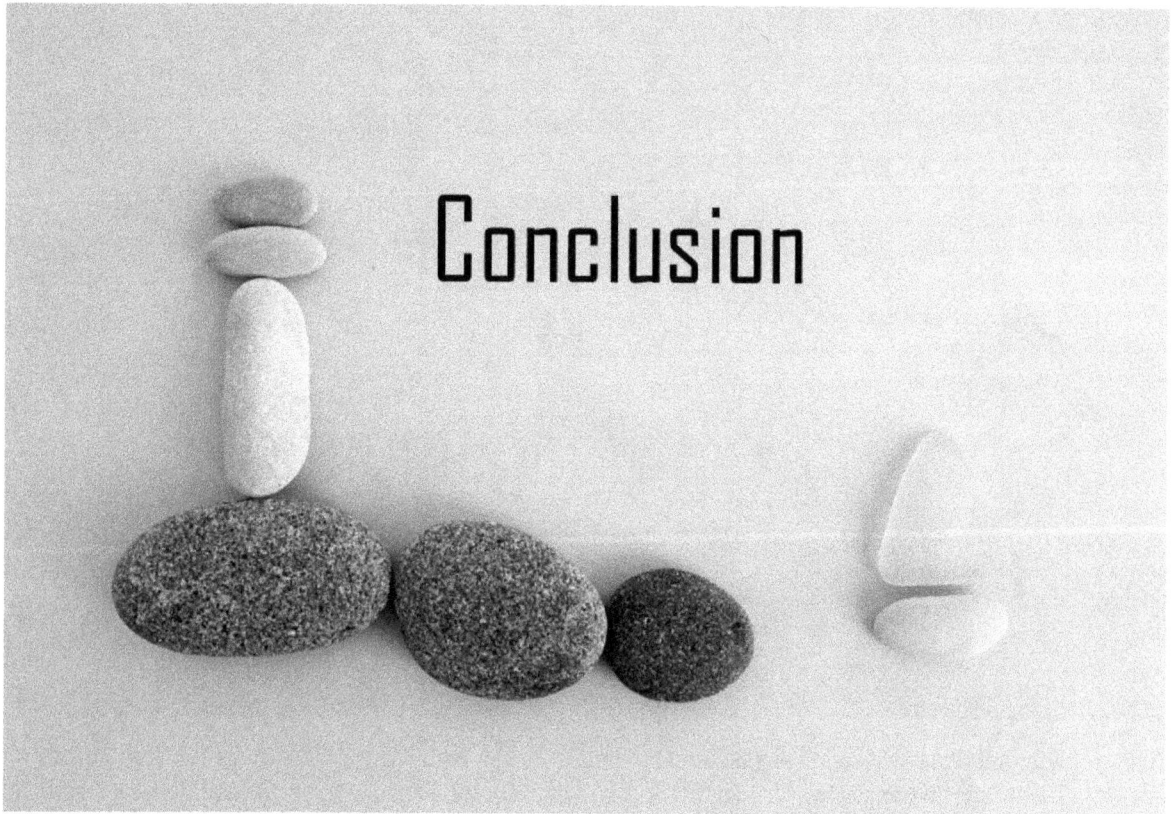

It is my hope that one or more of these tips helps you conquer your battle with chronic kidney stones. It is important you take care of yourself, have a good doctor, eat, sleep and hydrate properly to achieve the best quality of life possible.

You are worthy of self-care.

You are worthy of a life with as little pain and discomfort as possible.

Never believe you are a lost cause.

This world is full of a thousand possibilities. There is always hope.

You are not alone in this battle against your health.

Please take care of yourself. I promise you that you are worth it.

Thank you again for reading, <u>Chronically Stoned</u>.

May you find healing, hope and happiness.

Sincerely,

Winslow E. Dixon

Dedications & Acknowledgements

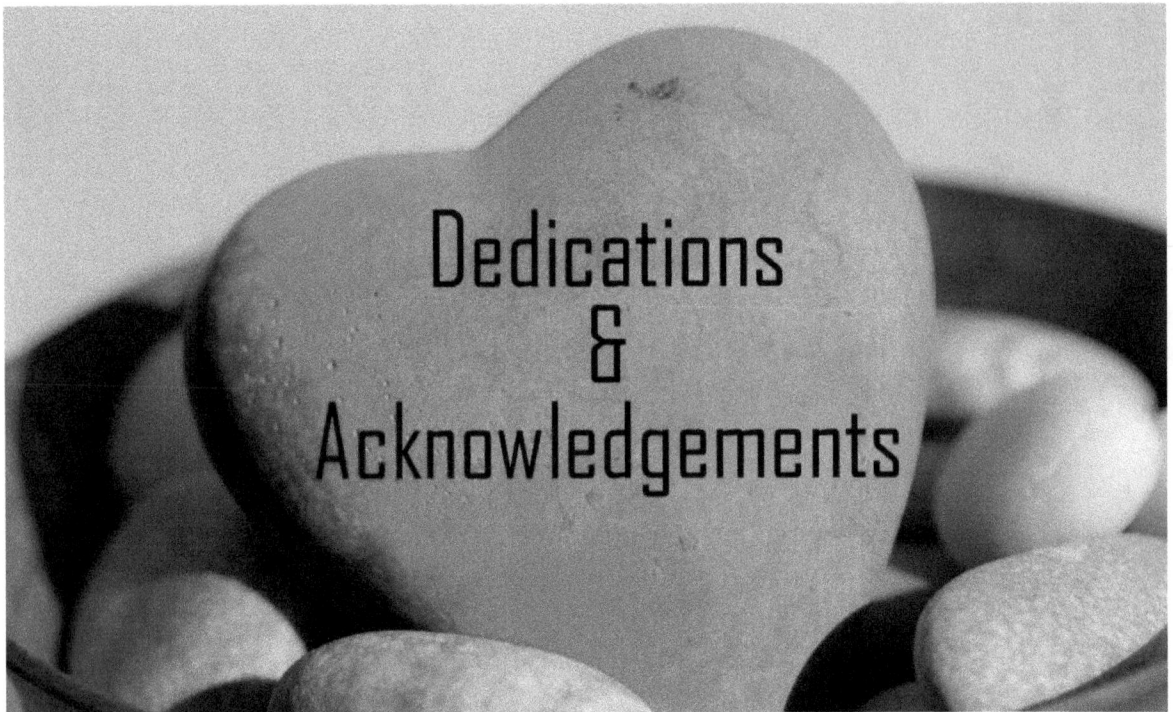

This book is first dedicated to the physician who diagnosed me with Medullary Sponge Kidney. For her privacy, I will refer to her as Dr. "V." Thanks to her, I can finally manage the congenital disease that went unnoticed through multiple medical systems. She took the time to look past my age and treat my symptoms as a suffering patient. Thank you so much Dr. "V" for your excellence in healthcare and how you are making a positive difference in humanity.

Secondly, this book is dedicated to Dr. Todd. His medical practice provides more than just healthcare, it is a ministry to those who are broken and suffering. Thank you for being such a compassionate doctor. I know Dr. "R" is bragging on you in heaven, even though we miss his brilliant, kind spirit on earth. Thank you for being a godly physician.

Thirdly, this book is dedicated to the people who keep me going. This life is difficult since my health failed and my career abruptly ended, and love is truly all that matters after all. Thanks to my family, friends and online supporters who have encouraged me.

Love is all that matters after all.

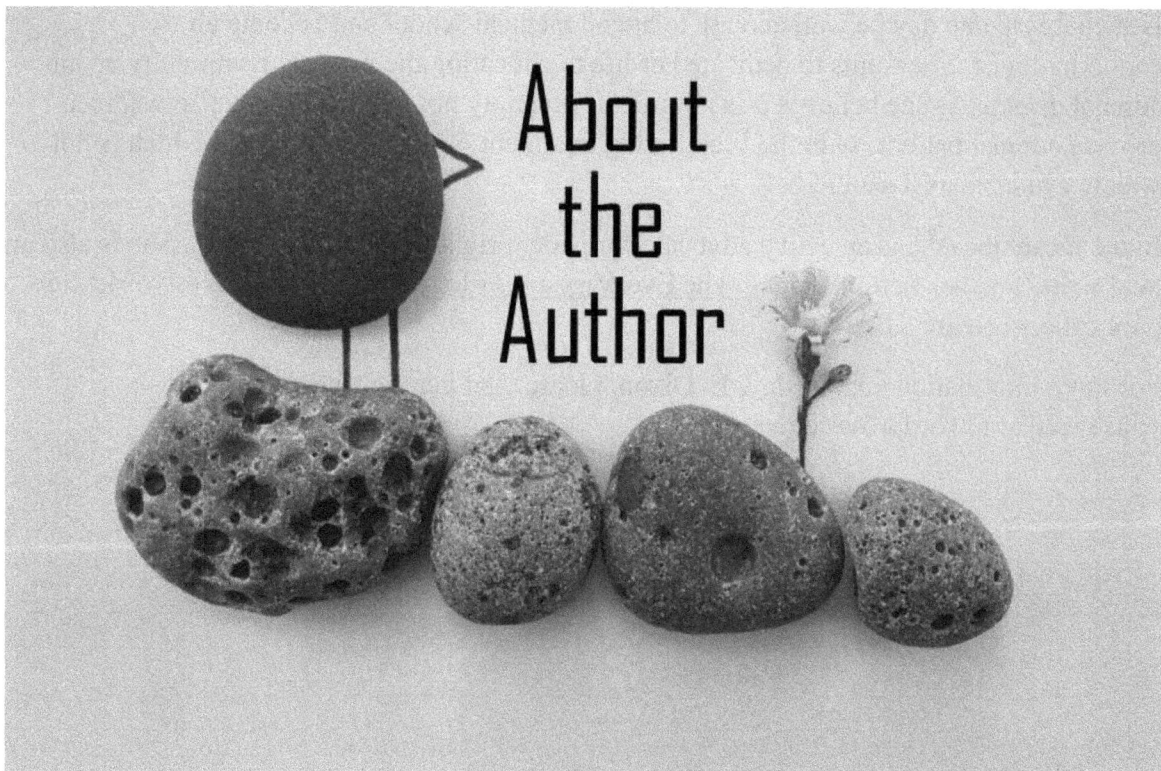

About
the
Author

Winslow E. Dixon started her young career in geriatrics. She specialized in Alzheimer's Disease and Dementia and worked as a resident enrichment director and memory care coordinator. She then continued her education, studying holistic health and nutrition.

She worked as a holistic health coach, aromatherapist, med-tech and medical thermographer. As a holistic health consultant through her business, Against the Grains LLC. She worked with those suffering from food allergies and helped clients establish rare disease diet protocols.

Upon her diagnosis of Medullary Sponge Kidney, Endometriosis and Addison's Disease, she was forced to find a new purpose. Winslow is now a published author, freelance writer and columnist. She volunteers her time as a political activist and patient advocate for those suffering with chronic illness, incurable pain, rare disease and disability. She is also a motivational speaker and has dedicated her life to spreading hope to those who are suffering through her patient advocacy organization, the Adrenal Alternatives Foundation. She is the author of the devotional journal challenge series, Arsenal of Arrows, the children's book written to explain disability to young children, The Shivering Sunbeam and the Peace by Piece 365 Day Inspirational Health Journal. All are available through Amazon, Kindle E-book and Barnes and Noble.

Her goal is to one day be well enough to attend medical school and become an endocrinologist. She wants to dedicate her life to educating the medical community about adrenal disease, as she believes it is not rare, it is simply not tested for. She also wants to provide adrenal patients with the life-altering treatment of the cortisol pump, which is not widely available as it should be.

In the meantime, she is an active advocate for patient rights and holistic health. She is also an avid writer and her fiction series – The EverVigilant Trilogy is in the process of worldwide publication- release TBA.

For more information on Winslow E. Dixon, please visit her website- winslowedixon.wordpress.com.

Sources

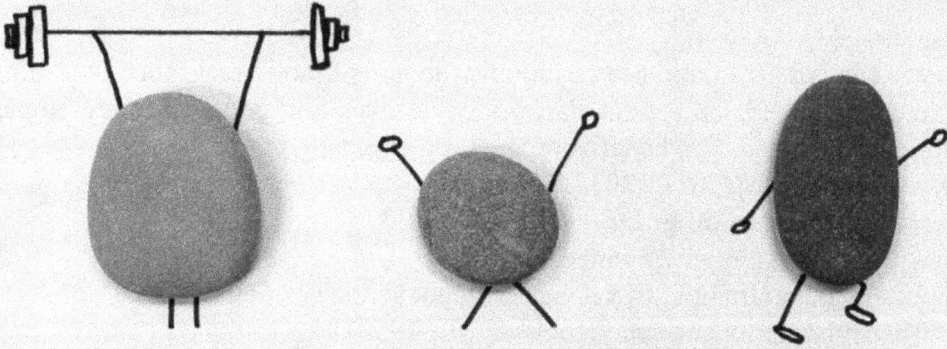

Drug Bank
Ethical Foods
Health Line
Medline Plus
National Center for Biotechnology Information
National Center for Disease Control
National Institute of Health Information
National Kidney Disease Foundation
Nutritional Anarchy
Second Opinion Newsletter
The Mayo Clinic
U.S National Library of Medicine
Urology Care Foundation

https://www.ncbi.nlm.nih.gov/pmc/articles/PMC1496869/
http://www.finallypainfreetx.com/history/fsm-microcurrents/
http://www.nutritionalanarchy.com/2014/04/14/citric-acid-comes/
https://www.medicalnewstoday.com/articles/154193.php
https://www.mayoclinic.org/diseases-conditions/kidney-stones/symptoms-causes/syc-20355755
http://ip-6.net/
https://www.cdc.gov/antibiotic-use/community/about/antibiotic-resistance-faqs.html
https://urology.wustl.edu/en/Patient-Care/Kidney-Stones/Surgery-for-Kidney-Stones
http://blog.vitaminworld.com/benefits-oregano-oil-supplements/
https://www.aafp.org/afp/2011/1201/p1234.html
https://www.drugbank.ca/drugs/DB00698
https://www.ncbi.nlm.nih.gov/pubmed/21170875
https://pubchem.ncbi.nlm.nih.gov/compound/tetracycline#section=Top
https://www.ncbi.nlm.nih.gov/pmc/articles/PMC3195018/
https://www.secondopinionnewsletter.com/Health-Alert-Archive/View-Archive/12052/How-to-treat-kidney-bladder-and-urinary-tract-infections-without-antibiotics.htm#
https://medlineplus.gov/clostridiumdifficileinfections.html#cat_92

For more information on the Frequency Specific Microcurrent Machine, visit the website-
https://frequencyspecific.com/

www.ingramcontent.com/pod-product-compliance
Lightning Source LLC
Chambersburg PA
CBHW051351290326
41933CB00043B/3435